ESSENTIAL OILS

A <u>7 Step Guide</u> For Cleansing Your Mind And Body Using The Earth's Natural Ingredients!

By Sophie Stevens

ISBN-13: 978-1793407474

Limits of Liability / Disclaimer of Warranty:

This information is for reference purposes only.
Statements are not intended as a substitute for professional healthcare
nor meant to diagnose, treat, cure or prevent medical conditions or
disease.
Every illness or injury requires supervision by a medical doctor or
alternative medicine practitioner.

The author and publisher of this book and the accompanying materials
have used their best efforts in preparing this program. The author and
publisher make no representation or warranties with respect to the
accuracy, applicability, fitness, or completeness of the contents of this
program. They disclaim any warranties (expressed or implied),
merchantability, or fitness for any particular purpose. The author and
publisher shall in no event be held liable for any loss or other damage,
including but not limited to special, incidental, consequential, or other
damages. As always, the advice of a competent legal, tax, accounting or
other professionals should be sought.

TABLE OF CONTENTS

INTRODUCTION 1

STEP 1 – UNDERSTAND WHAT ESSENTIAL OILS ARE........................5

STEP 2 – SIMPLIFYING AROMATHERAPY & ESSENTIAL OILS 7

    TERMS YOU NEED TO UNDERSTAND 7

STEP 3 – KNOW THE GENERAL SAFETY PRECAUTIONS 13

STEP 4 – HOW TO SHOP FOR ESSENTIAL OILS AND AVOID THE MANY PITFALLS 15

    HOW TO CHOOSE ESSENTIAL OILS.................................15

    USE THIS BOOK TO HELP CHOOSE YOUR PERFECT ESSENTIAL OILS 15

    HOW TO READ THE LABELS OF OILS 16

    LABELS TO LOOK FOR (HIGH QUALITY) 17

    LABELS TO LOOK OUT FOR (DUBIOUS QUALITY) 17

    SHOPPING FOR YOUR OILS 18

    STORING YOUR OILS 19

    WHERE TO BUY GOOD QUALITY ESSENTIAL OILS ONLINE 20

STEP 5 – LEARN THE METHODS OF USING ESSENTIAL OILS................23

    METHODS OF INHALATION 24

    TOPICAL APPLICATION..25

    DILUTING 26

    BLENDING 27

STEP 6 – FAST AND NATURAL HOME USES OF ESSENTIAL OILS..........29

    FASTEST NATURAL AIR FRESHENER.............................29

    INSECT BITE RELIEVER.......................................29

    SUNBURN RELIEVER & HEALER 29

    MATTRESS CLEANER AND DEODORISER............................30

    SKIN BLEMISH REMOVER 30

    NATURAL MOUTH WASH 31

    REDUCE ACNE AND BLOCKED PORES.............................31

STEP 7 – TOP 10 MUST HAVE BASE ESSENTIAL OILS: WHAT THEY ARE & WHAT THEY'RE GOOD FOR 33

    BASIL 33

CHAMOMILE 34

CINNAMON LEAF 36

EUCALYPTUS 38

GERANIUM 40

LAVENDER 42

LEMON 43

PEPPERMINT 45

ROSEMARY 47

THYME 49

BONUS – TOP 10 MUST HAVE ESSENTIAL OIL RELAXANTS: WHAT THEY ARE & WHAT THEY'RE GOOD FOR 53

BERGAMOT 53

CLARY SAGE 55

FRANKINCENSE 57

MARJORAM 58

NEROLI 60

ROSE 61

SANDALWOOD 63

SPEARMINT 65

TEA TREE 67

YLANG-YLANG 68

INTRODUCTION

Have you always been interested in essential oils and the natural benefits that they bring?

Do you prefer using natural methods for healing and rejuvenating your body rather than typical mainstream methods?

Have you dabbled in essential oils but haven't really discovered a simple way to understand how to use them and enjoy the natural benefits?

If you answer yes to these questions, then this guide will help you to discover the wonderful natural capabilities and properties of one of the world's oldest forms of healing.

It can sometimes be overwhelming learning each of the essential oils, like; which ones to buy, where to buy them, and how to use them.

The good thing is that when you do understand the fundamentals of essential oils, you can start using them to cleanse your mind and body regularly and feel completely rejuvenated.

This book is different to most references about essential oils because it goes through a step by step process for learning and understanding the 'essentials' before you start using them for maximum effect in your life.

Even if you have been using essential oils for years or have never used them at all but want to know where to start, this book will guide you in the right direction.

Here are some of the things you'll learn in this book:

- The essential terms and phrases you need to know

- How to buy essential oils, what to look for and where to buy the best quality

- How to be safe with essential oils – some essential oils are very intense and it is important to understand how to use them safely

- How to use essential oils – the different methods

- Discover some great natural uses of essential oils at home

- The top ten essential oils to have, what they are and what they're good for

STEP 1 – UNDERSTAND WHAT ESSENTIAL OILS ARE

Essential oils are the natural concentrated aromatic compounds extracted from the seeds, stems, petals, flowers, bark and other parts of different plants, but they also known as the plant's personality.

Essential oils are generally thinner than typical vegetable or animal oils but contain hundreds of organic properties which are packed full of healing properties.

They are also much stronger in their abilities because of their volatile organic compounds and also evaporate when left open.

So, what do essential oils contain?

In order for a plant to function, it requires hormones, vitamins and chemicals and these are what make up part of the essential oil from that plant.

The essential oil actually becomes the plants healing source to rejuvenate and heal the plant from damage. The essential oil also prevents evaporation and regulates the water content in a plant.

STEP 2 – SIMPLIFYING AROMATHERAPY & ESSENTIAL OILS

The key thing to consider is that aromatherapy is not intended to replace traditional medicine.

It is the application of natural medical treatments from plants organic healing compounds which have been used for thousands of years to rejuvenate and heal both plants and human beings.

The first step in understanding essential oils is by understanding the terminology.

Following terms and concepts will help you to understand Aromatherapy and essential oils which can sometimes be confusing to many people.

TERMS YOU NEED TO UNDERSTAND

Absolute Oils

Absolute Oils are different to essential oils because they are extracted through solvent extraction rather than steam distillation, which is the method for essential oils.

Solvent extraction is used for flowers or leaves that are too delicate to be extracted using steam distillation and this method produces a more volatile and concentrated oil which is called Absolute oil.

Carrier Oil

Carrier oils, which are also known as base oils or vegetable oils come from the fatty portion of a plant.

These oils are extracted from the pressing of seeds, nuts, vegetables or plants.

Some of the most common carrier oils are almond, coconut, jojoba and sunflower.

Carrier oils are essentially used to dilute essential oils and absolute oils before they are applied to the skin.

This is because if essential oils or absolute oils are applied to the skin directly, they can cause severe irritation or reactions.

Therefore, Carrier oils are used to 'carry' the oil

onto the skin.

In addition, Carrier oils retain moisture which prevents the essential oil from evaporating if not sealed.

Extraction

Extraction is where the oil molecules are removed from the plant 'matter'.

The extraction process is very important because it determines an essential oil's properties, benefits, and how it's used.

Although the extraction of essential oils may sound only to be of technical interest, it is one of the key points which determines the quality of the oil that is used.

The Most Common Methods of Extracting Essential Oils

The following are the primary methods of extracting essential oils:

- **Distillation By Steam** - This is where plant material is heated to form a vapor and the result is the essential oil when it cools down. Steam distillation is the preferred method over water distillation because it has less risk of damaging the components of essential oils because it is a faster and process. Distillation by Steam is one of the most common forms of essential oil extraction.

- **Solvent Extraction** - This extraction is used for plants that are more delicate in nature, like Rose or Jasmine, and cannot be used with other stronger methods of extraction. Essentially, this method has the plant exposed to different solvents to help extract the essential oil. The methods of solvent extraction are; enfleurage and maceration. Enfleurage is where the plant material is placed on a glass frame which is covered with an odorless fat or oil and then heated by the sun. Maceration is here the plant is soaked in heated purified oil. The plant matter is continually added until the oil is completely saturated by the plants essence.

Fragrance Oils

Fragrance oils can be made up partly of an essential oil but they are generally 100% synthetic.

This means that they contain many synthetic chemicals which can be toxic or harmful to your body.

Fragrance oils also have fixatives which help to extend the life of the oils aroma.

These should not be used in the same way as essential oil because Fragrance oils are specifically formulated to be ingredients in perfume, candles and soap.

Neat

In general, most essential oils are too strong to be used on the skin when it is undiluted.

This is why many essential oils have the warning: 'Do not apply neat'.

If the instructions say to apply 'neat', that means you can apply the essential oil undiluted.

There are not many essential oils that you can apply 'neat', but some of these exceptions are lavender and tea tree oil which can be applied directly to skin undiluted.

However, most essential oils will need to be diluted.

Organic Oils

Organic essential oils are becoming more and more popular as a choice for essential oil.

These oils must be certified organic just the same as organic food products.

Because they must be certified to be organic, they must have the Department of Agriculture (USDA) seal on the container.

Similar to food products, the plants which the essential oils are extracted from must not be subject to fertilizers, pesticides or preservatives.

STEP 3 – KNOW THE GENERAL SAFETY PRECAUTIONS

When using essential oils, it is really important to know and understand the safety precautions.

Also, prior to any use, if you have any questions, please consult your physician or a trained aromatherapist.

- **Never use an essential oil undiluted directly on skin or 'neat'** – Unless the container specifically states that the oil can be used 'neat'.

- **Always use a test skin patch** – This should be done before any first-time use of an essential oil.

- **Keep away from eyes**

- **Essential oils are highly flammable** - Use with extreme care around fire.

- **Keep essential oils in a locked cabinet** – This is to keep away from children.

- **Reduce doses for Babies and elderly people** – The dosage should be half that recommended for a healthy adult.

- **Do not use essential oils with chemotherapy**

- **Essential oils use for people with allergies to nuts** - People who have allergies to nuts must not use sweet almond or peanut carrier oils.

- **Essentials oils use for pregnant women (with caution)** – Consult your physician before any use.

STEP 4 – HOW TO SHOP FOR ESSENTIAL OILS AND AVOID THE MANY PITFALLS

HOW TO CHOOSE ESSENTIAL OILS

USE THIS BOOK TO HELP CHOOSE YOUR PERFECT ESSENTIAL OILS

There are 20 essential oils covered in this book and they are split into the top 10 base essential oils and top 10 essential oil relaxants.

These essential oils are a compilation by aromatherapists, retailers and manufacturers.

It is not the 'perfect' list for everyone but it is a great reference and start for you.

- **Step 1** - Choose five essential oils from the list of Top 10 Must Have Base Essential Oils that, when reading their properties and uses, feel in alignment with you.

- **Step 2** - Choose five essential oils from the list of Top 10 Must Have Essential Oil Relaxants, which fit as having the properties for fixing or healing the problem or situation you want to repair or correct.

- **Step 3** – Visit a health food store or drugstore, which sells essential oils, so you can sniff them to get a sense of which essential oils appeal to you and if there are any essential oils on your list which you don't like, cross it off. Go through your list and identify the ones that you like. You may only finish with one or two but that is fine.

HOW TO READ THE LABELS OF OILS

Before you decide to purchase essential oils, whether at a store or online, it's important understand how to read the labeling.

This is because there can be some subtle differences on a label which can have a substantial difference as to what is in the container.

LABELS TO LOOK FOR (HIGH QUALITY)

The phrases below denote high quality essential oil, which means if the container has one or more of the following, the quality will be high.

Therefore, you should look for these when you are shopping for your essential oils.

- 100% Pure Essential Oil

- Therapeutic Essential Oil

- No pesticides

- First distillation

- Undiluted & pure

- No additives

LABELS TO LOOK OUT FOR (DUBIOUS QUALITY)

The phrases below denote low quality essential oils or oils which may not be an actual pure essential oil.

It is suggested not to buy oils which have labels using any quotes from the above list.

- Rich in essential oil

- Blend contains essential oil

- Vitamin enriched oil

- Plant based oil

It is best to buy single essential oils, rather than blends or pre-mixed oils.

Because, this allows you to:

1) Monitor the level of dilution

2) Control the level of intensity of the aroma

3) Prolong the life span of the essential oils because they last longer in their 100% pure form

SHOPPING FOR YOUR OILS

When shopping around for your oils it is suggested you do the math.

This is because essential oils can be purchased at different stores ranging in different prices and quality.

It is suggested to compare the pricing of essential oils because they can vary a lot.

For example, high quality Rose Otto can vary from $250 to $800 per ½ oz. (15 ml) and depends on where you buy it from.

Also, prices can vary a lot depending on the country of origin.

The highest quality Sandalwood originates from India and costs around $150 per oz. (30 ml), whereas Sandalwood oil from Australia costs around $80 per oz.

Tip 1 - Only purchase essential oils if their bottle is dark blue glass or dark brown glass.

STORING YOUR OILS

Step 1 – Always buy good quality oils because they will last longer and make sure you are buying new stock, not old at your place of purchase.

Step 2 – Store the oils in a dark glass container and ensure it is airtight.

Step 3 – If you have a large quantity it is best to recant the oil by placing it into small containers as this reduces the amount of oxygen which the oil is subject to inside the container.

Step 4 – Place the oils in a cool dry place away from direct sunlight, 40 to 60 degrees Fahrenheit (5 to 20 degrees Celsius).

Step 5 – Only keep the essential oils for a maximum of 24 months.

WHERE TO BUY GOOD QUALITY ESSENTIAL OILS ONLINE

When people start looking to buy essential oils, they obviously want the best quality at the best price.

The problem is that it can be difficult to identify and differentiate good quality from bad quality; however the points explained previously should help you do this.

Below is a list of online stores that you can buy quality essential oils, and most of them ship anywhere in the world.

This list is based on research and a proven track record and quality, cost and delivery.

Simplers Botanicals - a good all round selection:

http://www.shopsimplers.com/

Auracacia - a large company which tests the quality of the oils before they sell them:

http://www.auracacia.com/auracacia/art.html

Floracopeia - a good company which visits and personally selects the oils:

http://www.floracopeia.com/

Veriditas Botanicals - great site for buying in bulk:

http://www.veriditasbotanicals.com/oils_lav.html

New Directions – very popular and renowned site:

http://www.newdirections.com.au/content.php?p=home-home-campaigns

Sydney Essential Oil Co. – certified organic:

http://www.seoc.com.au/

STEP 5 – LEARN THE METHODS OF USING ESSENTIAL OILS

Essential oils are incredibly versatile and can be integrated into your daily life in many different ways.

There are two main methods of using essential oils:

- **Inhalation** – This method is where the oil enters the body via inhalation through the nose or mouth. When the molecules of the essential oil enters the blood stream through the lungs, the brain and nervous system is affected which in turn releases hormones to different areas of the body.

- **Topical Application** – This method generally means the essential oil is diluted with a carrier oil and then applied directly to the skin. This process means the essential oil can also enter the blood stream but through the skin. In the same way, the brain and nervous system is affected releasing hormones to different areas of the body.

Fundamentally, essential oils are drawn to a particular hormone or body part which it is most effective.

Different oils are more effective in their rejuvenation and healing to different areas of the body and this is why it is important to understand the capabilities of each oil.

METHODS OF INHALATION

- **Diffusing** – This method is where oil is diffused into the air by a vaporizer, humidifier or room spray etc. The essential oil is combined with steam or water to be diffused into the air and is then breathed.

- **Cupping** – This method is where drops of oil are placed in the palm, and the hands are then cupped over the nose and inhaled gently and deeply. It is a more intense form of allowing the oils molecules to enter the body.

- **Sniffing** – This is directly sniffing from an open viral and is commonly used because it is the fastest method of allowing the essential oils molecules to enter the blood stream.

- **Perfume** – This is wearing a perfume which has a mixture of an essential oil with a carrier oil.

TOPICAL APPLICATION

- **Full body massage** – This must be done with an essential oil that has been diluted correctly with a carrier oil. It is one of the most popular methods of application because of the relaxed delivery of the essential oil into the body. The diluted oil is massaged on certain point of the body which the specific essential oil is known provide healing properties to have maximum effect.

- **Bath** – This method allows for a more diluted topical application where the essential oil is added to the bath water.

- **Application Mixer** – This is where the essential oil is mixed into applications like body lotions, soaps, shampoos and conditioners.

DILUTING

A general guide for diluting essential oils is the following:

1% dilution for children and the elderly – Add 15 drops of essential oil to one ounce of carrier oil in a dark glass bottle. Seal and shake to mix the oils.

2.5% dilution for general, whole-body massage – Add six drops of essential oil to one ounce of carrier oil. Seal and shake to mix to the oils.

5% dilution for concentrated, local massage – Add 30 drops of essential oil to one ounce of carrier oil. Seal and shake to mix the oils.

Tip – When adding essential oils to a bath, it is best to dissolve the essential oil into honey (50/50) as this will stop the essential oil from clogging in one spot.

BLENDING

Blending simply means the mixing together of essential oils and carrier oils.

To get the best results, you will need to do some experimenting.

By experimenting you will discover more about the properties of the individual oils and how they work together.

STEP 6 – FAST AND NATURAL HOME USES OF ESSENTIAL OILS

FASTEST NATURAL AIR FRESHENER

Step 1 – Place a bowl of boiling water in the room you want to scent

Step 2 – Add 1-8 drop of an essential oil of your choice

Step 3 – Wait a few seconds and the whole room will be filled with a fragrant scent

INSECT BITE RELIEVER

Step 1 – Add 2-3 drops of Lavender oil with 1 tablespoon of carrier oil

Step 2 – Apply to the insect bite on the skin

SUNBURN RELIEVER & HEALER

Step 1 – Place 4 oz. of distilled water into a spray

bottle

Step 2 – Add 10 drops of lavender oil

Step 3 – Spray on burnt area, which will relieve the pain and start the healing process

MATTRESS CLEANER AND DEODORISER

Step 1 – Add 2-3 drops of an essential oil of your choice to a cup of baking soda

Step 2 – Sprinkle over the mattress and leave it for 1-2 hours

Step 3 – Vacuum up

SKIN BLEMISH REMOVER

Step 1 – Place 1 drop of Tea Tree oil on to the blemish

Step 2 – Watch the blemish start to disappear

NATURAL MOUTH WASH

Step 1 – Place 1 cup of Aloe Vera juice into a shakable bottle

Step 2 – place ½ cup of water into the bottle

Step 3 – Add 2 teaspoons of baking soda into the bottle

Step 4 – Add 20 drops of peppermint oil

Step 5 – Mix well. Use as a normal mouth wash.

REDUCE ACNE AND BLOCKED PORES

Step 1 – Add 3-4 drops of Tea Tree oil to warm water

Step 2 – Lean over the bowl with a towel over your head

Step 3 – Stay there for 10 minutes and let the steam fill your face

Step 4 – Do this process every 3-4 days

STEP 7 – TOP 10 MUST HAVE BASE ESSENTIAL OILS: WHAT THEY ARE & WHAT THEY'RE GOOD FOR

BASIL

What is Basil oil?

Basil oil is extracted from the herb Ocimum basilicum, which is an aromatic herb and has yellow green leaves.

This oil is also known as 'sweet basil' or 'holy basil'.

It has a watery viscosity with a pale yellow color.

The aroma is a sweet, light mint with licorice tones. Basil oil the most similar to Rosemary oil, however it is less intense.

What is Basil Good For?

- **Anti-spasmodic**: This oil is great for muscle and digestive spasms.

- **Pain Relief:** An excellent treatment for

menstrual cramps and tension.

- **Digestion:** It has carminative properties which is used for treating indigestion, constipation, stomach cramps and flatulence.

- **Mental fatigue:** Works to alleviate mental stress and fatigue to aids quick thinking and decision making.

What are the Precautions?

- **Do not use during any stage of pregnancy, sensitive skin or children.**

- **Do not over-use** – Do not use more than 6 drops to 1/2 oz. of carrier oil.

CHAMOMILE

What is Chamomile?

Chamomile is a flowering plant in the daisy family and is native to Europe and Asia.

The oil has a deep blue color and provides a sweet

and herbal fragrance.

The dried flowers from the Chamomile plant are used to make the well-known Chamomile tea, which has relaxation properties.

Chamomile has a very calming effect which means it is used a lot in massage oils.

What is Chamomile Good For?

- **Anti-inflammatory:** This oil is great for skin rashes, blisters and allergies.

- **Pain Relief:** Chamomile is an analgesic and is helpful for relieving pain, muscles spasms, headaches and cramping.

Chamomile can be used to treat:

- Indigestion

- Anxiety

- Insomnia

- Canker sores

- Conjunctivitis

- Crohn's disease

- Diarrhea

- Eczema

- Hemorrhoids

- Menstrual pain

- Migraines

What are the Precautions?

- **Do not use if the color is not blue** – If your Chamomile oil has begun turning green, from a blue color, it should not be used.

CINNAMON LEAF

What is Cinnamon Leaf Oil?

Cinnamon leaf oil is extracted from the leaves of Cinnamomum zeylanicum.

This tree grows to a height of 45 feet and bears small, green leaves with white flowers and little purple berries.

Cinnamon leaf oil is a yellow, watery substance and has a warm, rich and spicy aroma.

What is Cinnamon Leaf Oil Good For?

- **Brain Tonic:** This oil boosts the activity of the brain and helps remove brain tension.

- **Vaporizer:** Cinnamon is great in a diffuser, and a great treatment for colds and viruses.

- **Blood Circulation:** This oil is great for people with low blood circulation as it will increase blood flow and warm the body.

- **Arthritis:** Cinnamon leaf oil is also a great treatment for arthritis pain.

What are the Precautions?

- **Avoid using on sensitive skin.**

- **Do not over-use** – do not use more than 3 drops with a bath and no more than 3 drops to 1/2 oz. of skin lotion or massage oil.

EUCALYPTUS

What is Eucalyptus Oil?

Eucalyptus oil is extracted from the leaf of the Eucalyptus tree which is also known as Tasmanian blue gum.

It is native to Australia and has spread to other parts of the world including South Africa and Europe but the highest quality Eucalyptus oil comes from Australia.

This tree is tall and evergreen, and can grow to 100 feet high.

The leaves are dark green but produce oil which is a light yellow color.

Its aroma has a strong and distinct woody and balsamic scent and is one of few essential oils which increases its intensity with time.

What is Eucalyptus Good For?

- **Respiratory problems:** Eucalyptus oil is great for treating problems like sore throat, nasal congestion, bronchitis, sinusitis and the common cold. Medical studies have actually published findings which show Eucalyptus oil to produce faster improvement in patients with respiratory problems.

- **Anti-septic:** This oil is great for healing wounds, burns and cuts by providing anti-septic properties.

- **Muscles soreness:** Eucalyptus oil can be massaged into the skin can provide pain relief because it has analgesic and anti-inflammatory properties.

- **Insect repellent:** This oil is great for preventing and treating insect bites.

- **Mental Exhaustion:** This oil is has a refreshing and stimulating effect and helps with feelings of exhaustion and stress.

What are the Precautions?

- **There are no precautions for Eucalyptus oil.**

GERANIUM

What is Geranium Oil?

Geranium oil is extracted from the all parts of the Geranium plant, including its stalks, leaves and florets.

The fragrance of this oil has a floral aroma with a hint of mint and is light green in color.

It is a great substitute for Rose oil because it is less expensive.

What is Geranium Good For?

- **Antiseptic:** Its antiseptic qualities detoxify the lymph system.

- **Hemorrhages:** Geranium oil causes the

blood vessels to contract to stop the blood flow and increases the clotting of the blood.

- **Skin Scars and Blemishes:** This oil facilitates blood circulation just below the surface of the skin and help distribute melanin to help fade and vanish skin scars and blemishes.

- **Cellulite:** Added to massage oil, geranium is effective in reducing cellulite.

- **Deodorant:** It's also a good personal deodorant, as well as room freshener and insect repellant.

What are the Precautions?

- **There are no precautions for Geranium oil.**

LAVENDER

What is Lavender Oil?

Lavender oil is one of the most useful essential oils you can have.

It is extracted from the lavender bush and the highest quality Lavender comes from England and France.

Lavender is generally a colorless but can have hints of green and yellow.

It has a floral, sweet aroma with a hint of wood and balsamic.

Lavender is used a lot in skin lotions, perfume, and household cleaners.

What is Lavender Good For?

- **Muscle relaxant:** This oil is great for muscles tension or muscle spasms and also helps to relieve headaches.

- **Pain Relief/Antiseptic:** Great for relieving

pain and sunburn and prevent infections. It can be used as an insect repellant and therefore is very good for inspect bites.

- **Allergy Reliever:** Lavender is one of the few essential oils that can be applied 'neat' and is great for treating acne and skin allergies.

What are the Precautions?

- **Do not use during preliminary stages of pregnancy** - Lavender should not be used during the first trimester of pregnancy.

- **Must be used in a carrier oil on children and infants.**

LEMON

What is Lemon Oil?

Lemon oil is extracted from the rind of the common lemon which is one of the most popular fruits in the world.

The extraction process is done using the form of cold-pressing from the rind of the lemon.

Its aroma is a clean, lightly sweet scent similar to fresh lemon rind and is pale yellow in color and has many health benefits.

What is Lemon Oil Good For?

- **Insomnia:** Lemon oil assists in sleep and helps with insomnia.

- **Stomach disorders:** Lemon oil neutralizes stomach acid and helps with heartburn discomfort.

- **Low Immune System:** It is useful for limiting the spread of bacterial infections, colds, and sore throats.

- **Hair Care:** Lemon oil is great for removing dandruff and building strong shiny hair.

- **Skin care:** When added to massage oil or lotions, Lemon oil is great for dull, oily skin, dark spots, and varicose veins.

- **Low Immune System:** Lemon oil has a very
  high vitamin content which helps to increase
  the body's immune system.

- **Weight Loss:** This oil is great for assisting in
  losing weight.

What are the Precautions?

- **Do not use on skin direct with sunlight -**
  Lemon oil is photosensitive and therefore
  should not be used on the skin within 24
  hours of being expose to sunlight.

- **Do not use on sensitive skin.**

- **Use Sparingly –** Do not use more than 3
  drops in bath water or ½ oz. in massage oil
  or body lotion.

PEPPERMINT

What is Peppermint Oil?

Peppermint oil is extracted from the peppermint

plane and is a cross between water mint and spearmint.

The oil is a pale green color and has a penetrating smell with a hint of grass and camphor.

It has a stronger smell than spearmint.

Peppermint oil is one of the oldest oil dating back to ancient Egypt and Greece.

It has a menthol content of 50% - 85% which gives it a minty fragrance.

What is Peppermint Good For?

- **Indigestion:** It is very helpful for digestion when putting a few drops of peppermint oil in a glass of water and taking after meals. It also helps relieve irritable bowel syndrome, constipation, vomiting or nausea.

- **Dental Care:** This oil is great for removing bad breath due its antiseptic properties and helps teeth and gums prevent germs.

- **Migraines:** This oil can be effectively used

for treating chronic migraines by diluting in a carrier oil and lightly massaged on a forehead and neck.

- **Respiratory:** This oil contains menthol which helps in clearing the respiratory tract.

What are the Precautions?

- **Use with caution on sensitive skin -** Peppermint oil must not be used 'neat' and should only be used in a carrier oil.

- **Do not use on children under 5 years old.**

ROSEMARY

What is Rosemary Oil?

Rosemary oil is extracted from a bushy shrub called Rosmarinus Officinalis, which has silver-green leaves.

Rosemary oil is one of the most popular essential

oils because of its versatile benefits.

Rosemary oil is a colorless oil and has a sweet herbaceous fragrance which gives it a fresh aroma.

Rosemary oil is most commonly used to stimulate hair growth and boost mental activity because it is the strongest essential oil for aiding brain function.

What is Rosemary Good For?

- **Hair Care:** Rosemary oil is used in shampoos and lotions because it stimulates hair follicles which helps the hair to grow longer and stronger. Place a few drops of Rosemary oil in shampoo, conditioner or water will help to stimulate the scalp, remove dandruff and revitalize the hair.

- **Mouth Care:** This oil is a disinfectant and helps to eliminate bad breath.

- **Booting Mental Activity:** Rosemary oil diffused in the air helps to clear the mind and stimulate creative thinking and concentration.

- **Room Aroma:** This oil has a mesmerizing aroma and is commonly used in room fresheners, candles and perfumes. Combining Rosemary oil and water and spraying around will help remove bad odor from a room.

What are the Precautions?

- **Do not use during pregnancy at any stage.**

THYME

What is Thyme?

Thyme oil is extracted from the common herb, Thyme, which has small green leaves and white flowers.

There are more than 150 species of Thyme, where the strongest in Red Thyme which is characterized by its orange-brown-red color.

All varieties of Thyme generally have the same

aroma, but Red Thyme is the most intense with a sweet, spicy, woody fragrance.

What is Thyme Good For?

- **Anti-septic:** Great for fighting infection, either bacterial or viral.

- **Low Energy:** Thyme oil stimulates production of red blood cells, which increases oxygen throughout the body. This oil also helps to restore strength and stamina, especially for chronic fatigue sufferers.

- **Anti-spasmodic:** Thyme oil is fantastic for reducing the unwanted spasms causing coughs, cramps and aches.

- **Anti-Rheumatic:** This oil increases urination to help remove toxins and also stimulates circulation to help remove toxins like uric acid from the blood stream, which helps with rheumatism, arthritis and gout.

What are the Precautions?

- Do not use during pregnancy during any stage.

- Do not use in cases of high blood pressure.

- Do not use Red Thyme in massage oil or bath water due to its strength.

BONUS – TOP 10 MUST HAVE ESSENTIAL OIL RELAXANTS: WHAT THEY ARE & WHAT THEY'RE GOOD FOR

These oils have all been selected as the 10 most commonly used essential oils which have the best relaxant capabilities.

As an additional set of oils to the top 10 base essential oils, these relaxants are all excellent in their own way and will complement any set of essential oils.

BERGAMOT

What is Bergamot?

Bergamot oil is extracted from the plant Citrus Bergamia, which is mainly grown in Italy.

The oil is extracted from the peel of the fruit and produces a sweet, refreshing aroma even though the fruit is sour to taste.

Bergamot oil is a green-yellow color and is used in

perfumes and also Earl Grey tea and has a calming effect.

What is Bergamot Good For?

- **Anti-biotic:** This oil is great for killing germs and viruses in relation to eczema, herpes, acne and oily skin. It is also great for urinary tract infections.

- **Anti-depressant:** Bergamot is a mild sedative and stimulates hormone secretion to help increase circulation relieve stress and anxiety and promote positivity.

- **Digestive Problems:** Bergamot activates secretions o digestive acids to promote and assist in the digestive process and regulates the intestines.

Bergamot is usually inhaled to treat anxiety.

What are the Precautions?

- **Do not use 'neat'** – This oil must not be

used undiluted on the skin. It must be used with a carrier oil or lotion.

- **Do not use within 12 hours prior to sun exposure** – Most Bergamot oil is photosensitive, which means it should not be used on the skin within 12-14 hours of being exposed to the sun. Few Bergamot oils are able to be used with sunlight, however they must be labeled with 'Bergaptine free'.

CLARY SAGE

What is Clary Sage?

Clary Sage oils is extracted from the leaves of the Clary Sage plant (Salvia sclarea) of the Labiatae family.

The method of extraction is steam distillation from the leaves of the plant.

The oil has a musky and floral aroma and promotes revitalization.

What is Clary Sage Good For?

- **Anti-depressant:** This oil helps with anxiety and depressive feelings because it produces a very positive feeling.

- **Anti-bacterial:** Clary Sage Is great for preventing the spread of bacteria and kills the bacteria especially for intestinal and urinary tract infections. It is also great for treating dandruff.

- **Deodorant:** Clary Sage is used in many deodorants and perfumes and can be diluted and made as a great natural deodorant.

- **Anti-spasmodic:** This oil is great for relieving muscle spasms and cramps and spasmodic coughs.

What are the Precautions?

- **Do not use with alcohol** - Use with alcohol or drugs may have side effects.

- **Do not use during pregnancy or with infants.**

FRANKINCENSE

What is Frankincense?

Frankincense oil is extracted from the small Boswellia Sacra tree which grows in India, Africa and the Middle East.

The oil is taken from the resin of the tree and produces a woody and balsamic aroma.

It is a popular oil in cosmetics and incense burners and has been used for hundreds of years in Christian religions.

What is Frankincense Good For?

- **Skin Care:** This oil is great for restoring skin which is dry and wrinkly. It also helps with skin scars and stretch marks.

- **Astringent:** Great for strengthening teeth and gums and hair roots and contracts blood vessels to prevent hair loss and wrinkles in old age.

- **Sedative:** Franki9ncense is an effective

sedative and promotes mental peace and relaxation.

- **Tonic:** This oil also boosts the body's nervous system and respiratory system to increase health.

What are the Precautions?

- **There are no safety precautions or warnings for Frankincense.**

MARJORAM

What is Marjoram?

Marjoram oil is extracted by steam distillation from the Marjoram plant which is evergreen.

The oil is colorless and has a woody and spicy fragrance and is use in many perfumes but is most known for its sedative properties.

What is Marjoram Good For?

- **Analgesic:** This oil is great for reducing cold and fever symptoms and tooth aches and does not have any real side effects.

- **Anti-spasmodic:** Marjoram is very effective in treating all types of spasms.

- **Sedative:** This oil promotes a relaxing and calming effect on the mind and body especially for people who have experienced grief or extreme sadness.

What are the Precautions?

- **Use Marjoram in small amounts** – This oil should not be used in large amounts due to its sedative strength.

- **Do not use during pregnancy** - Marjoram must not be used at any time during pregnancy.

NEROLI

What is Neroli?

Neroli oil is a plant extracted oil which is produced from the fragrant white flower blossoms of the bitter orange tree native to Italy.

It is a pale yellow oil and has a fresh floral aroma.

The oil is extracted by water distillation instead of steam distillation due to the delicate nature of the blossoms and is one of the most expensive essential oils you can buy.

What is Neroli Good For?

- **Skin Care:** Neroli oil great for rejuvenating all skin types because it regenerates the skin cells. It is found in many skin care products, massage oils and bath oils because of its skin toning abilities.

- **Anti-depressant:** This oil is great for treating chronic anxiety or feelings of major disappointment and helps with depression and post-traumatic stress because it regenerates optimism and confidence.

- **Mind Rejuvenation:** This uplifting oil helps with shyness and promotes creative thinking.

What are the Precautions?

- **There are no safety precautions or warnings for Neroli.**

ROSE

What is Rose Oil?

Rose oil is extracted from the damask rose which grows across Bulgaria, Turkey, Russia, India and China.

It is extracted from the petals of the flower and can range in color from light pink to a strong deep red.

One of the most expensive essential oils and most common is Rose Otto which is produced by water distillation and costs between $600 and $1,500 per oz.

On the other hand, Rose Absolute, which is distilled with an alcohol solvent, and has a much stronger fragrance than Rose Otto costs half the price.

However, the two essential oils are more or less the same properties and capabilities.

What is Rose Good For?

- **Anti-depressant:** Rose oil helps with depression, grief, anger, fear and stress.

- **Menstrual Problems:** This oil can also be an effective treatment for premenstrual cramps and premenstrual stress as well as menopause.

- **Skin Care:** Rose oil is used in many skin care products and helps with mature or dry skin.

What are the Precautions?

- **Do not use during the first trimester of**

pregnancy - Rose oil should not be used during the first three months of pregnancy.

SANDALWOOD

What is Sandalwood Oil?

Sandalwood oil extracted from the inner areas of the sandalwood tree.

This tree's wood is heavy, yellow and fine-grained unlike many other trees; it retains its fragrance for decades.

Because of this, Sandalwood oil is the longest lasting of the essential oils and its aroma becomes better over time.

It is also one of the most expensive essential oils because of its rarity and is commonly found in designer fragrances as the base note.

The aroma of this oil is a striking and woody and has a sweet, fresh odor.

The purest and highest quality Sandalwood oil comes from India, however, the tree has become endangered and this contributes to its higher expense.

Sandalwood oil from Australia is about half the price of sandalwood oil from India and is considered to be very similar in its properties and capabilities.

What is Sandalwood Good For?

- **Mind Clarity:** Sandalwood oil is wonderful for relaxing, balancing the mind and reducing confusion.

- **Anti-septic:** This oil is great for treating bronchitis and laryngitis.

- **Skin Care:** Sandalwood is also great for treating acne and scalp conditions, like dandruff.

What are the Precautions?

- **Do not apply 'neat' to the skin** - Sandalwood oil should not be applied undiluted (neat) directly to the skin.

- **Use it sparingly** – Sandalwood has a very persistent fragrance and should be used sparingly.

SPEARMINT

What is Spearmint Oil?

Spearmint oil is extracted from Mentha spicata, which is spear shaped green leaf flower that grows to about 3 feet tall.

Spearmint has a similar aroma to that of peppermint oil, however is slightly sweeter and is pale yellow-green in color.

It is not as popular as peppermint oil but this essential oil is far less harsh for use with children.

It is most commonly known as a flavor in chewing gum and candy because it is sweet, cooling and calming.

What is Spearmint Good For?

- **Pain Relief:** Spearmint oil is great for chronic headaches or chest pain because it helps you sweat and cool down. It also helps with sore muscles. To relieve sore muscles, add 20 drops of spearmint to 3.5 oz. of water in a spray bottle and spray on the sore muscles.

- **Disinfectant:** This oil has strong anti-bacterial properties and can be used as a disinfectant for wounds.

- **Teeth Whitening:** Spearmint oil is fantastic for teeth whitening and also helps keep gums healthy.

- **Facial Skin Care:** This oil clears and tightens pores and leaves the skin feeling firm.

What are the Precautions?

- **Do not use around eyes even when**

diluted in a carrier oil.

TEA TREE

What is Tee Tree Oil?

Tee Tree oil is extracted from the leaves of Melaleuca alternifolia, which has medium green to yellow leaves and is a plant native to Australia.

It is a pale yellow color, nearly colorless, and has a spicy aroma similar to nutmeg.

This oil is one of the most medicinal of the essential oils and is able to fight bacteria, viruses and fungi.

What is Tee Tree Good For?

- **Anti-bacterial:** Tea Tree oil can be applied undiluted (neat) directly to the skin to treat rash, athlete's foot, cold sores, herpes, insect bites, head lice and acne.

- **Vaginal Yeast Infection:** This oil is great for treating vaginal yeast infection. This can be done by taking a warm Tea Tree bath.

- **Cold and Flu:** Tea Tree oil can be used to alleviate cold symptoms and a sore throat with steam inhalation.

What are the Precautions?

- **Use in moderation** – This oil must be used in moderation. For example, no more than 2% in a carrier oil and no more than 4 drops in a bath.

- **Use with caution with skin application** - This oil is strong and can irritate sensitive skin.

YLANG-YLANG

What is Ylang-Ylang Oil?

Ylang-Ylang oil is extracted from the Cananga tree's yellow flowers which is found in Indonesia.

Ylang-Ylang is a pale yellow clear oil with an sweet, almond and floral aroma.

The quality of Ylang-Ylang is determined from that the flowers were picked and the distillation process, where the best time to pick these flowers is in the early morning.

There are three grades of Ylang-Ylang oil:

Ylang-Ylang Extra – Is typically distilled for a short duration.

Ylang-Ylang I, II and III – Once Ylang-Ylang Extra is collected; the distillation process then continues then stops. III is equal to three distillation processes.

Ylang-Ylang Complete – is obtained from a complete, uninterrupted distillation process.

What is Ylang-Ylang Good For?

- **Anti-Depressant:** Ylang-Ylang helps with overcoming sadness, anger and anxiety.

- **Aphrodisiac:** This oil helps with impotence when used around the abdomen and groin area.

- **Anti-Septic:** Protects from infections from bacteria, virus and assists in faster healing.

- **Stress Reduction:** This oil is a great pre-sleep stress reduction method. This can be simply done by adding 4 drops in bath water and also helps with insomnia.

What are the Precautions?

- **Do not use for long periods of time** – Do not use this oil for long periods as it may result in headache or nausea.